Essential Oils:

DIY Body Lotions and Recipes With Essential Oils For Healthy Weight Loss

Table of Content :

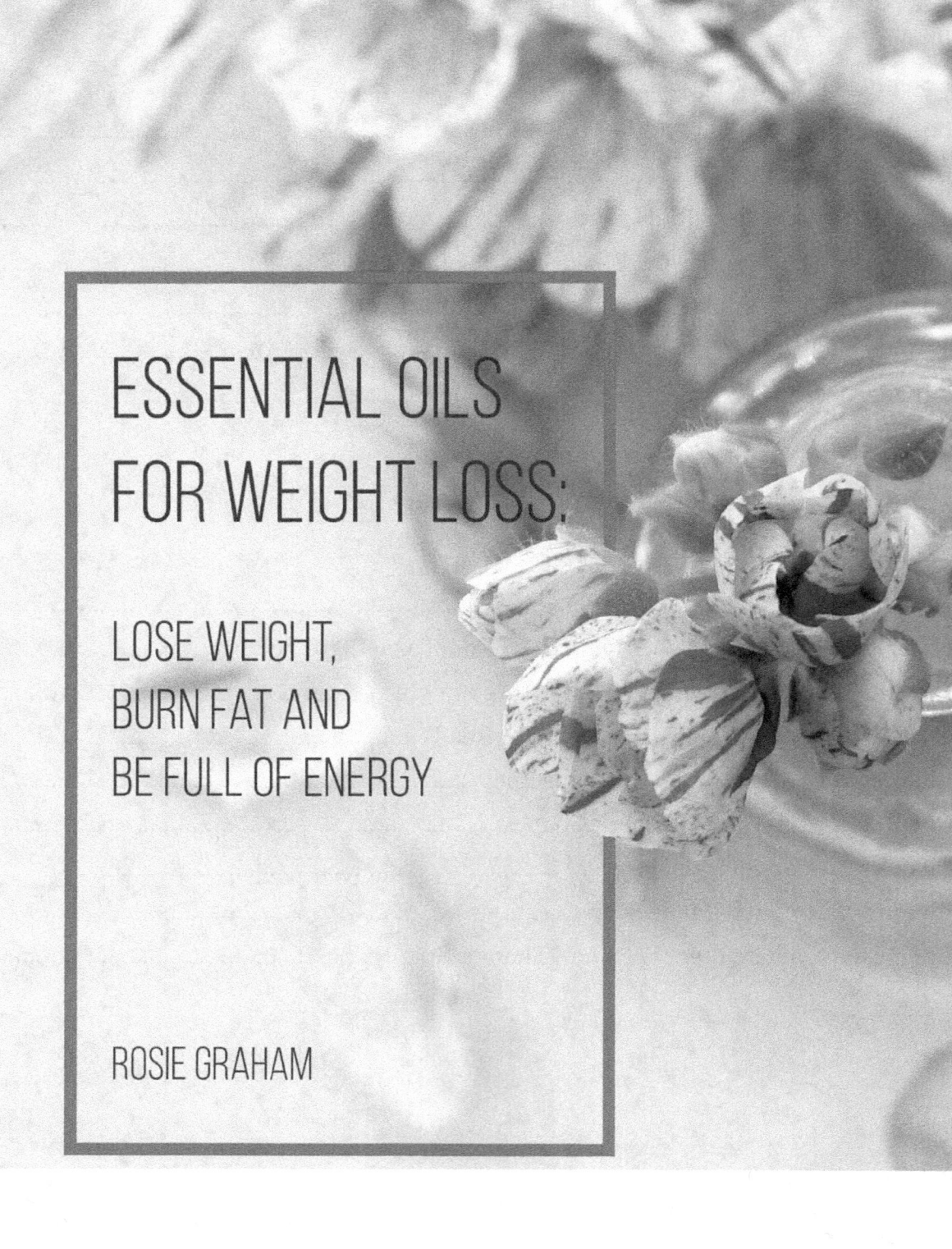

ESSENTIAL OILS
FOR WEIGHT LOSS:

LOSE WEIGHT,
BURN FAT AND
BE FULL OF ENERGY

ROSIE GRAHAM

Essential Oils for Weight Loss

Lose Weight, Burn Fat and Be Full of Energy

Introduction

Essential oils have been a recent trend among people whether celebrities or not who are interested in losing some weight. Weight loss is good whether for health purpose or the sake of good looks.

Essential oils are natural yet powerful. Also, they are easier to follow compared to diets that alter regular feeding style. The research on essential oils is ongoing with many exciting discoveries already made.Apart from the fact that essential oils are effective for weight loss, they are also useful in achieving balanced emotions, appetite control as well as a good scent for your body.

In this book, you'll find a short discussion about how essential oils work, why they work, some essential oils and how to use them as well as some essential oils recipes that you can make from the comfort of your home. That's a major advantage of essential oils the ease of preparation.

This book also mentions how you can work essential oils into your bracelet and necklace using ceramic diffuser beads to hold the scent of your essential oil all day.

I wish you success on your journey to weight loss using essential oils.

Chapter 1 – Why Essential Oils work

Different cultures from various parts of the world have known about the benefits essential oils have some of which are therapeutic and can heal. The abilities of the essential oil have been in full use for over 6000 years some to countries and empires like the Greeks, Chinese, Romans, Indians and so much more.

The essential oils are from various parts on a plant or tree. There are essential oils that they extract from the root, stem, bark, flowers and fruits. And for this reason, the essential oils in themselves will have different features that distinguish them from others.

A good example will be the essential oils that are known to have strong anti-inflammation properties, while others can be insecticidal or anti-microbial. In this light, there are also some essential oils that fat burning capabilities or help to curb cravings or unnecessary appetite.

How Essential Oils Work For Weight Loss

Your brain contains parts that are responsible for putting your body in the best physical shape and the right mental state, such that the when you stimulate these parts of the brain properly there are some have a general positive on you as an individual and this practice is known as *Aromatherapy*.

The human nose contains receptors that can perceive trillions of different kinds of smell, and they also have a crucial function of communicating to the amygdala and hippocampus in the brain, which are essential places where you keep memories and information.

Now for every inhalation of essential oils, study suggests that the amygdala and hippocampus are greatly affected such that they, in turn, influence our emotional and physical states almost instantly and directly, some of which are our motivation, mood, stress and sleep.

Even though presently there is no substitute for a healthy diet and regular exercising to help with weight loss, essential oils can go a long way to help with your weight loss target.

So eventually whether or not you fight a constant battle with cravings, low moods, slow metabolism, fatigue and emotional eating, essential oils can be that missing ingredient you need to achieve your weight loss target.

Chapter 2 – How to Use Oil Essentials for Weight Loss

Research by the Smell and Taste Treatment along with the Research Institute of Chicago resonated around the fact that continually inhaling culinary smell throughout the day (3-6 times)can go a long way in suppressing the desire to eat or taste anything especially when hungry.

Furthermore, the research advised that you should continue to change the essential oil you use across the day as this will help you to avoid the problem of familiarity with the essential oil, this will also bring a higher degree of efficiency.Here are some essential oils that can help you lose weight

Types of Essential Oil and How to Use Them

Cinnamon Essential Oil

It won't be strange to find that most people with diabetes use this oil.A study done in 2013 indicated that cinnamon "has anti-parasitic, anti-oxidant, anti-microbial and free radical scavenging properties".And also that it tends to reduce serum cholesterol and blood glucose.

The study also indicates that cinnamon oil has excellent abilities in stabilizing blood glucose level and Glucose Tolerance Factor (GTF) in the body, this is essential because blood sugar levels could also lead to over-eating, lower energy levels, weight gain, sugar craving and even irritability.By adding cinnamon oil to food, it can help in slowing down the rate by which glucose flows into your bloodstream, and this will help you in achieving your weight goals in the long run.

Cinnamon leaf oil contains eugenol, and this alters the neurosensory perceptions and also affect the way we taste and smell food, and this will help to reduce food craving and also stop overeating.

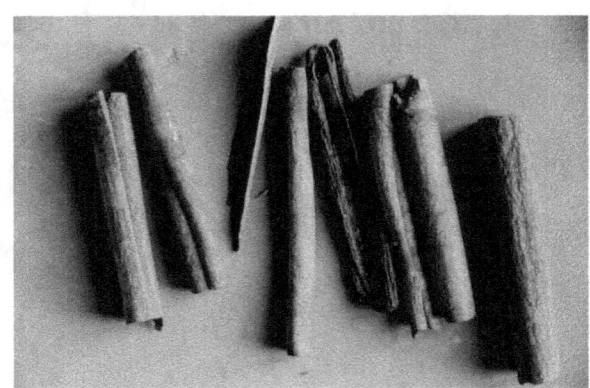

Using Cinnamon Essential Oil for Weight Loss:

- By drinking it: the FDA recommends that the cinnamon oil is safe to take directly internally, but it is advisable that you buy therapeutic-grade cinnamon essential oil.Therapeutic-grade cinnamon essential oil is 100% pure and toxin and addictive free.

  Therapeutic-grade cinnamon essential oil is unfiltered and undiluted. You can also add 1 to 2 drops of cinnamon oil into warm water (about a teacup) with a little touch of honey (raw honey would work fine and better) to help in the fat loss.If you do this daily, it helps in reducing cravings. To curb late night food craving, it is advisable that have it before a meal or when the craving for food surfaces. You can also add cinnamon oil to your oats, baking or smoothies.

- Inhale directly: to prevent overeating before a meal or whenever a sudden carving sets in, you can inhale some cinnamon oil straight out of the bottle. As you do this regularly, it could go a great deal in improving your mood and make you fuller. It is advisable for emotional eaters.

- Apply topically: mix one to two drops of cinnamon oil with either of coconut oil or jojoba oil. After you do this, apply by rubbing it on your chest and wrist.

- Diffuse: put drops of cinnamon oil into your diffuser as this will not only give the house a great smell but will also help to stimulate a good mood.

Lemon Essential Oil

Lemon essential oils are known to be extracted from the lemon skin and containing the compound limonene, which makes lemon oil a characteristic fat dissolver.A recent report recommended that when joined with grapefruit oil, lemon oil supported lipolysis (separating of body fats) making it a "suppression in body weight gain."

Lemon oil additionally detoxifies and take out poisons in the body that can be stored in the fat cells, slow down parasites in the intestines, and improve digestion.

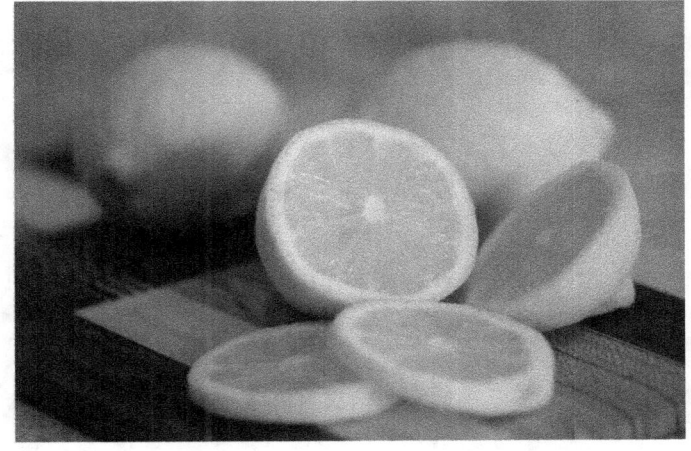

<u>Using Lemon Essential Oil for Weight Loss</u>

- Mix 2 drops of lemon oil to a glass of water in the morning and drink, this will help in detoxifying. It also supports digestion.

- Inhale the lemon directly from the bottle or soak cotton balls into the container and inhale directly from the cotton balls, this will curb cravings for food and decrease overeating.

- Blend the lemon oil with oils like coconut oil (carrier oil) and massage the mixture into areas that contain cellulite build-up.

Bergamot Essential Oil

Nervousness, gloom and low moods are frequently the major causes with regards to emotional eatingGiving in to your cravings may help light up your state of mind in the short term span yet over the long haul it just prompts sentiments of blame and low esteem, particularly when you heap on the pounds.

An ongoing 2015 investigation inferred that simply breathing in bergamot oil for 15 minutes can help your state of mind as well as decrease cortisol (a pressure hormone), that has a negative impact on fat loss.

In a recent report, 237 members with hyperlipemia (elevated amounts of fat in the blood) were given a fresh extract of bergamot orally for 30 days, and the investigation demonstrated that they could diminish blood cholesterol levels and altogether help in the reduction of blood glucose.

Bergamot contains polyphenols (a similar compound found in green tea), and it can push the body to dissolve fat and sugar normally. The sweet citrus aroma of bergamot oil gives you a high sense of feel, causing you to unwind and also smother cravings and control emotional eating.

Bergamot also has an enormous amount of limonene (additionally found in grapefruit oil and lemon oil), bergamot oil can burn fat. As indicated by University Health News, "D-limonene goes about as a gentle appetite suppressant and counteracts weight gain."

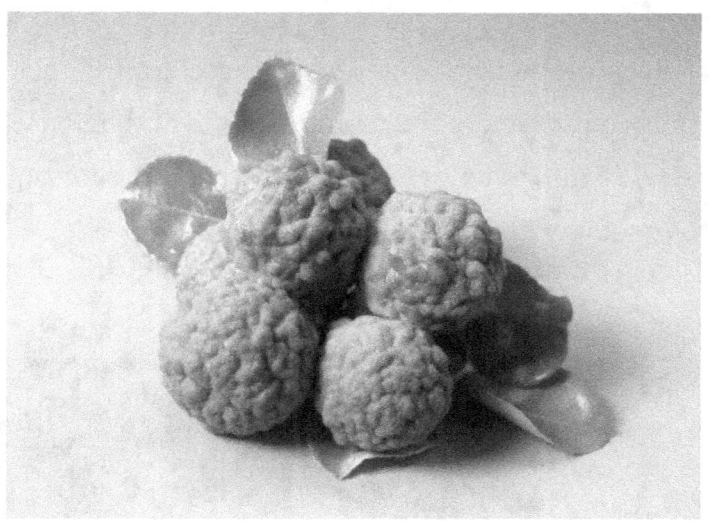

Using Bergamot Essential Oil for Weight Loss

- Inhale the oil directly or use a cotton ball soaked in oil, this scent of limonene will help to suppress cravings which in turn helps you to lose weight.

- Add this essential oil to your shower and cover the drain, inhale the scent to get the maximum benefits which keep you refreshed and in the right mind to lose weight.

Frankincense Essential Oil

Frankincense oil is gotten from the native of a tree local to Somalia, in Africa, and is fantastic for calming uneasiness and low inclinations that can trigger the need to eat more to food to feel satisfied.

Wealthy in sub-atomic structures called sesquiterpenes, that can cross the blood-cerebrum boundary, frankincense oil can ease the negative impacts of both uneasiness and misery.

Frankincense oil can encourage digestion by accelerating the flow rate of bile and gastric juices which in turn influences the metabolic rate and helps weight reductionIt can likewise stimulate peristaltic movement which enables food to move quickly through the digestive organs, improving digestion.

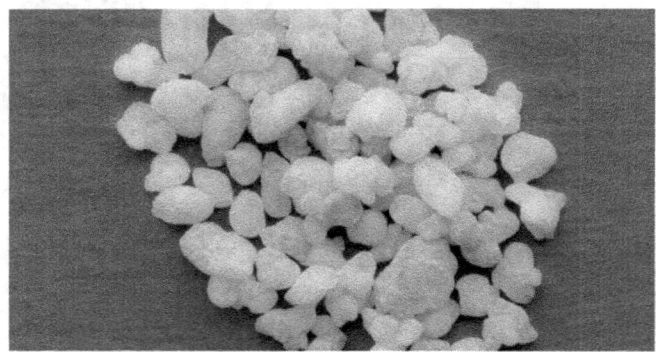

How to Use Frankincense Oil

- Inhaling a few deep breaths of frankincense essential oil will help subdue hunger pangs and induce a calm feeling.

- Add a few drops (2-3) frankincense oil to your diffuser and allow its sweet aroma fill the air surrounding you, this will help to lead away anxious feeling and calm your mind leaving you with lesser cravings.

Jasmine Essential Oil

Jasmine essential oil extracted from the sweet-smelling jasmine bloom, a research study recommends that the scent of Jasmine is very calming.

Jasmine oil has been utilized for quite a long time to cure uneasiness, low sex drive, sleep deprivation and misery; furthermore, research demonstrates that jasmine can calm despondency and elevate your mood.

This trait makes it a phenomenal fundamental oil to use if you are attempting to get in shape and can't control cravings and fell the need to turn to food when you're feeling low or experience difficulty sleeping off at night (which can prompt late night immense consuming of food).

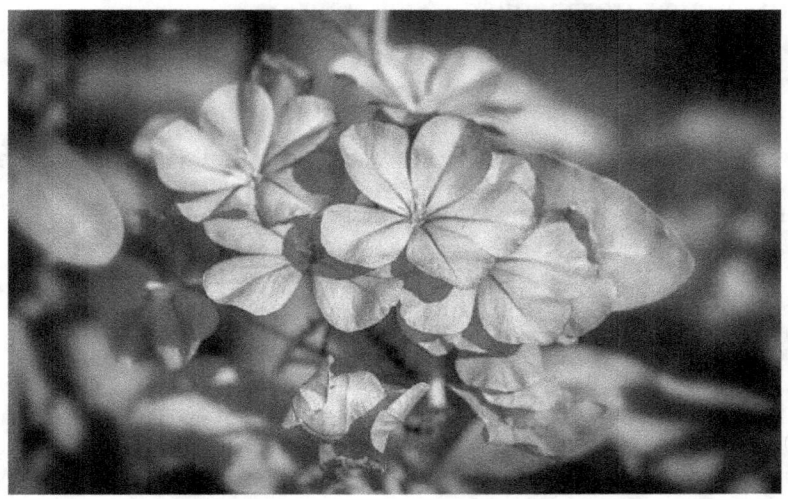

<u>Using Jasmine Essential Oil for Weight Reduction</u>

- Inhale jasmine essential oil before taking a meal, and it will help to calm your senses to prevent you from over-eating. You can also go further to put a few drops of this essential oil on your handkerchief and carry it along with you all day, inhaling from time to time.

- Combine about 2-3 drops of jasmine and about 4-5 drops of grapefruit oil in you diffuse which will send a citrusy scent that will keep you in a good mood and help relax the nerve that causes food cravings.

Orange Essential Oil

Orange oil can control appetite and reduce overeating. It contains Vitamin C and furthermore has a cancer prevention agent benefit. The sharp citrusy aroma is additionally a ground-breaking mood enhancer and can help many experiencing discouragements.A research study from Japan's Mei University demonstrated that orange oil helped members decrease their energizer medicine consumption.

There are uncountable investigations which demonstrate that depression prompts weight increase and this one shows its direct relationship with really causing a higher hazard of obesity

.By utilizing essential oils like orange oil and different oils referenced above, you can lift your mood, feel much improved, and be less enticed to use food to feel better.

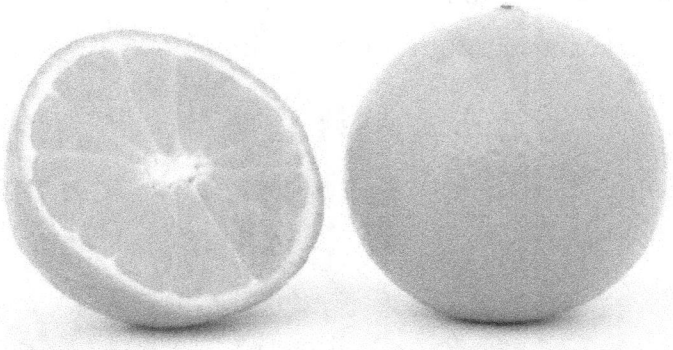

<u>Using Orange Essential Oil for Weight Reduction</u>

- Drink a glass of water containing 1-2 drops of orange oil before you take a meal to help reduce cravings and stop overeating

- Dab a cotton ball in few drops of oil and inhale directly to keep you perked up and stimulate your senses to keep you from overeating.

Rosemary Essential Oil

The rosemary essential oil originates from rosemary sprigs through steam refining. Rosemary essential oil is a solid, ground-breaking oil that can complete something significantly beyond flavor meat and potato dishes.

As indicated by a recent report directed in Japan, rosemary oil can diminish cortisol (the pressure hormone) levels in spit, and this is significant as high cortisol levels relate to dangerous health conditions, for example, hypertension and heart disease.

High cortisol levels lead to elevated feelings of anxiety, which can prompt emotional eating and weight gain. Keeping your cortisol levels low is critical to lessening your feelings of anxiety which will cause less emotional eating and keep your weight in charge.

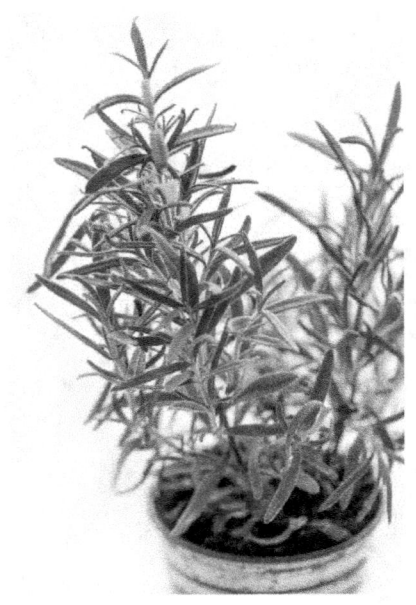

Using Rosemary Essential Oil for Weight Reduction

- When you feel stressed inhale rosemary oil for about 3-5 minutes taking as many deep breaths as you can help in reducing cortisol levels and help your waistline.

Grapefruit Essential Oil:

Grapefruit is well known for helping people lose weight for decades. The grapefruit diet also called the Hollywood Diet since the 1930s.

According to research, when mice are with food containing a lot of fat for three months, the mice were given grapefruit juice to drink gains up to 18% less weight than those that take water.

Grapefruit is gotten from the fresh rind, grapefruit essential oil is an excellent appetite suppressant, detoxifier and helps to prevent water retention in the body and to bloat as it also helps in dissolving fats.

It is a fact that the rind from which the oil originates contains a high concentration of nootkatone, which is a component which is responsible for activating AMP-activated protein kinase (AMPK). AMP-activated protein kinase makes the body reduce fat accumulation and use up sugar which in turn results to weight loss.

In a nutshell, AMP-activated protein kinase is stimulated by grapefruit oil which leads to more fats burned away.In another research, rats are also exposed to grapefruit essential oil 3 times weekly for fifteen minutes, and it led to reduced body weight and food intake in the rats

Limeone is another vital component of grapefruit oil that causes lipolysis (i.e. a process where the body dissolves proteins and fats), this allows reducing appetite and body fat.

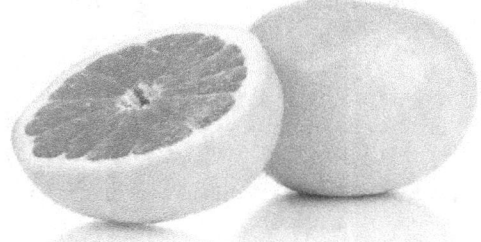

Using Grapefruit Essential Oil for Weight Loss

- Diffuse: put a few drops of grapefruit oil into your diffuser especially when you want to stop late night snacking.

- Dink it: put two drops of therapeutic-grade grapefruit essential oil in water, one glass full. You must ensure that you drink this every morning as soon as you wake up, this will help in increasing the reaction, detoxifying the body by flushing out toxins, increasing fat loss and helps in maintaining your weight.

  After taking a meal, you could also drink the grapefruit oil as it helps to digest food.

- Inhale directly: if suddenly, you are craving, the fresh scent of grapefruit oil can do a lot. You can decide to inhale it directly from a bottle, or you can also add a few drops into a cotton ball and inhale deeply. The scent of grapefruit makes the parasympathetic gastric nerve (the body mechanism that allows ghrelin-induced feeding) to relax.

- Apply topically: you could apply it by rubbing it on your wrist, temples, chest and also under your nose as it helps to curb appetite and also control carvings.

- Reduce cellulite: the oil is also effective in preventing water retention and also activates the lymphatic system. It contains a powerful anti-inflammatory enzyme called bromelain that allows and stimulates the breakdown of cellulite.

  That is why many producers use grapefruit in many cellulite creams. If you want to reduce the cellulite naturally, try the chemical-free blend written below.

Grapefruits Essential Oil All Natural Cellulite Cream:

Ingredients:

15 drops grapefruit oil

Glass Jar

1/2 cup coconut oil

Instructions:

In a blender, blend the coconut oil with the grapefruit oil and store the mixture in a glass jar. Rub onto the part of the skin that has cellulite and massage for 5 minutes daily.

Ginger Essential Oil:

Ginger as an anti-inflammatory is necessary for weight loss as it reduces inflammation which allows a more efficient absorption and digestion of food nutrients.In ginger, a compound called gingerols. Study indicates that this compound called gingerols reduces inflammation in the intestines and therefore makes the overall absorption of nutrients more efficient as it also helps in preventing diseases.

As long as your goal is to lose weight, the ginger essential oil will assist in absorbing the minerals and vitamins that you need to improve your cellular function and energy. You can be sure that it helps you to achieve your weight loss intentions.

A research done in 2013 showed us that ginger oil "possesses antioxidant activity as well as significant anti-inflammatory" properties and in about a month improved enzyme levels in the lab mice's blood had noticeably reduced chronic inflammation.

Another research in 2014 also indicated that to reduce obesity that is caused by increased fat diet, supplementing with ginger will help a great deal. The study also concluded that ginger is a "promising adjuvant therapy for the treatment of obesity."

Ginger oil helps a lot if you are having problems with fat belly. An article published in 2004 in the Biological Pharmaceutical Bulletin indicates that ginger is a cortisol suppressant.

Blood cortisol levels can be caused by High cortisol level which is also as a result of a hormonal imbalance and stressful lifestyle, and this could also push the body's natural metabolism out of place.

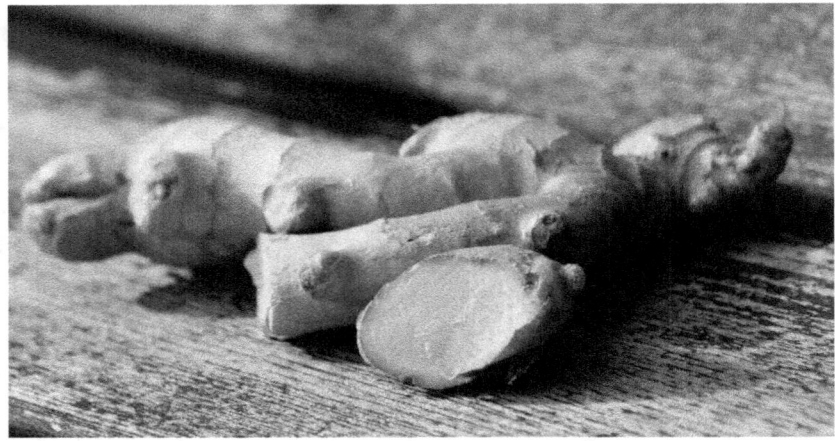

Using Ginger Essential Oil for Weight Loss:

- By drinking it: FDA authorizes that ginger oil has no side effects or dangers when taken directly internally, but it is best and advisable that you use therapeutic-grade ginger oil for internal use. You can also include one to two drops of ginger oil into a warm glass of water and also a squeeze of lemon juice and some honey (raw honey would be advisable).

- Inhale directly: you can also inhale the smell of the ginger oil straight out of the bottle as it serves as a great pick-me-up and also reduces unnecessary appetites and food cravings.

Peppermint Essential Oil

Peppermint has been in use for quite a long time, and it has been used to treat indigestion and particularly when joined with caraway oil has it can help to loosen up stomach muscles and swelling.

The cooling therapeutic compound in peppermint oil, menthol, is phenomenal for improving digestion, expelling gas from the stomach and intestines and easing an irritated stomach.

Menthol can impact neurosensory discernments to change how we taste and smell nourishment, avoiding cravings for sugary sustenances, other sustenance cravings and curbing gorging.

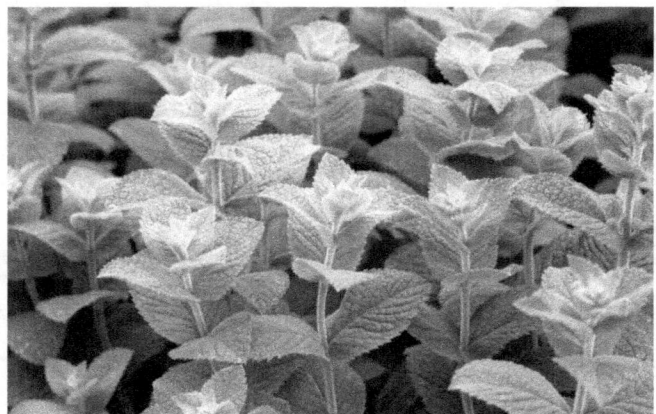

Using Peppermint Essential Oil for Weight Loss:

- Inhale it: You can decide to inhale it directly from a bottle, or you can also add a few drops into a cotton ball and inhale deeply.

The smell of the peppermint can take your mind away from food giving you a sense of relaxation. If you do this before eating, it can help prevent overeating and reduces your appetite.

According to the FDA, it is safe to take internally. About 1 to 2 drops of peppermint essential oil could also be added to a glass of water and taken before a meal as it helps to suppress and reduce appetite.

It is advisable that you buy and use therapeutic grade peppermint essential oil. Therapeutic grade peppermint essential oil is 100% pure and toxin and additives free. You can be rest assured that therapeutic grade peppermint essential oil is undiluted and unfiltered.

- Diffuse: by adding a few drops of peppermint essential oil into your diffuser especially when you feel like snacking. The mint scent is capable of curbing depression and will also go a long way in getting you energized.

Sandalwood Essential Oil

It is also advisable that you eat when you are stressed out if you are an emotional eater. Sandalwood essential oil also helps in reducing depression and creates a sense of calm. It has an exciting woody scent.

It also has a therapeutic effect on that part of the brain that dictates primal emotions like hunger, pleasure, anger and more. It makes a balance in your emotions, and thus food will not be something you turn to feel good. When this is done, you are a step closer to achieving your weight loss goal.

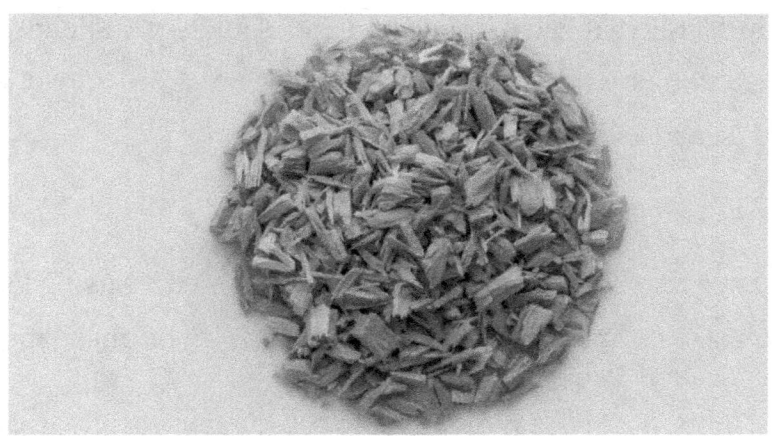

Using Sandalwood Essential Oil for Weight Loss:

- Inhale it: You can decide to inhale it directly from a bottle, or you can also add a few drops into a cotton ball and inhale deeply. The smell of the sandalwood can take your mind away from food giving you a sense of relaxation.

- Apply topically: you could apply it by rubbing it on your wrist and ankle as it helps to curb appetite and also control carvings after a long day's job.

- Diffuse: by adding a few drops of sandalwood essential oil into your diffuser especially when you feel like snacking.

Lavender Essential Oil

Each of the essential oils works in various ways in fighting weight loss. Some works in preventing fat accumulation, some others aids digestion, while others reduce appetite and lots more.

A significant factor that causes obesity today is anxiety and depression. "Feelings such as guilt, sadness, anger, and anxiety can often trigger series of overeating" says the National Centre for Eating Disorder.

Study indicates that stress and anxiety can be calmed by using lavender essential oil. Lavender oil also reduces that trigger that causes emotional eating.

Lavender oil also reduces cortisol level. Cortisols level has to do with the stress hormone that allows the body to retain fat which makes it tougher to lose weight.

A research done in 2010 by International Clinical Pharmacology indicates people using 80 mg per day of lavender showed less anxiety than those using a placebo. Another study done in 2013 shows that when rats are exposed to lavender for seven days inhibited depression-like behaviors and anxiety.

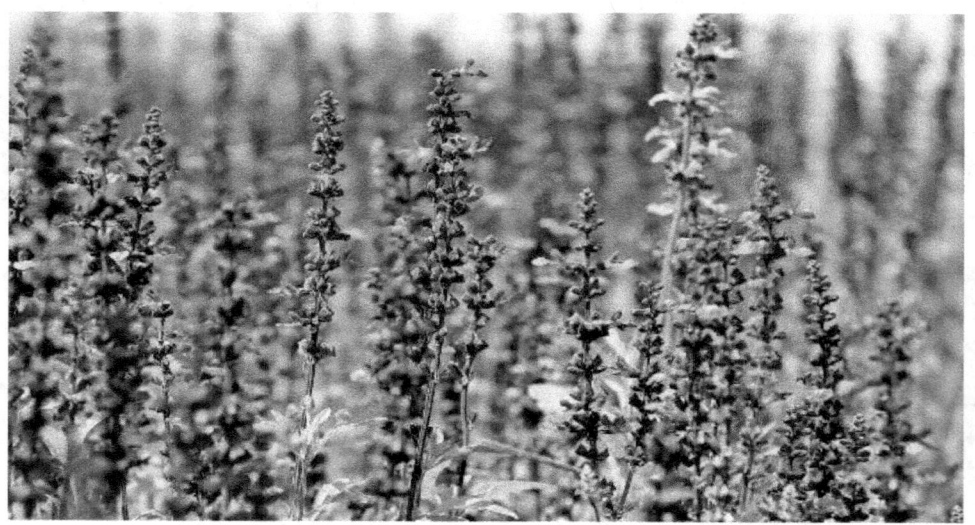

<u>Using Lavender Essential Oil for Weight Loss:</u>

- You can decide to inhale it directly from a bottle, or you can also add a few drops into a cotton ball and inhale deeply.

  The fresh scent enters the brain's center of emotion called amygdala and can take your mind away from food giving you a sense of relaxation and by adding a few drops of sandalwood essential oil into your diffuser especially when you feel like snacking.

  The pleasant aroma wafts around in the air and helps in reducing food temptation and anxiousness.

Chapter 3 – Essential Oil Recipes for Weight Loss

Weight Loss Capsule

Ingredients:

12 drops fractionated (liquid) coconut oil

2 drops lemon essential oil

2 drops peppermint essential oil

Vegetarian gel capsule (empty)

2 drops grapefruit essential oil

Instructions:

- ✓ Mix the coconut oil with the essential oils in a small container very well.
- ✓ Put the mixture into the capsule using an eyedropper.
- ✓ Use a capsule before breakfast daily to help with weight loss.

More recipes can be used at once to prepare capsule worth a week or even more.

Appetite – Curbing Diffuser Blend

Ingredients:

1 drop spearmint essential oil

3 drops grapefruit essential oil

1 drop ylang-ylang or rose essential oil

3 drops lemon essential oil

Instructions:

- ✓ Mix all the essentials oils in the ingredient list for this recipe in a diffuser.

- ✓ Before having a meal, diffuse one to two hours.

Essential Oil Boosted Drinking Water

Ingredients:

2 liters of drinking water

8 drops grapefruit essential oil

Instructions:

- ✓ Put the grapefruit essential oil into the 2 liters of water.

- ✓ To assist with the weight loss and also to eat less, take the 2 glasses of grapefruit mixed with water an hour or two hours before meal.

Weight Loss Foot Rub

Ingredients:

5 drops cypress essential oil

4 drops lavender essential oil

2 teaspoons carrier oil of choice (argan, avocado, coconut, sesame, sweet almond, jojoba, grapeseed, macadamia)

3 drops juniper essential oil

4 drops basil essential oil

8 drops grapefruit essential oil

Instructions:

- ✓ In a small beaker, mix all the ingredient above.

- ✓ Gently rub on the feet before going to bed (you could add water to increase efforts towards weight loss)

- ✓ You can use More quantity can be used for more than one use.

Weight Loss Massage Oil

Ingredients:

30 drops lemon ESSENTIAL OIL

40 drops grapefruit ESSENTIAL OIL

30 drops rose ESSENTIAL OIL

30 drops geranium ESSENTIAL OIL

1 ounce fractionated (liquid) coconut oil

Instructions:

- ✓ In a glass bottle, mix all of the ingredients above.

- ✓ Use it on your body taking your while taking bathing to help speed up weight loss, and you could use a professional massage session.

Citrus Anti-Cellulite Cream

Ingredients:

2 tablespoons witch hazel

10 drops lemon essential oil

30 drops grapefruit essential oil

¾ cup of coconut oil

2 tablespoons beeswax

Instructions:

- ✓ In a small bowl, mix the essential oils with the witch hazel.

- ✓ In a double boiler using medium heat, dissolve the beeswax and the coconut oil making sure that they melt.

- ✓ When you complete the above, remove from heat and mix the oils with witch hazel then stir gently to mix thoroughly.

- ✓ Put the result of the above step in a glass jar and wait to cool.

- ✓ Cover the glass tightly and store in a cool place. Wait for about 3 hours before making use.

Better Than a Tummy Tuck Cream

Ingredients:

15 drops geranium ESSENTIAL OIL

¼ cup beeswax (grated)

15 drops lavender ESSENTIAL OIL

15 drops grapefruit ESSENTIAL OIL

1 cup extra virgin olive oil

15 drops frankincense ESSENTIAL OIL

⅛ cup vitamin E oil

1 cup rose water

<u>Instructions:</u>

- ✓ In a double boiler, add all the ingredients above apart from the rose water and the essential oils.

- ✓ Place the mixture on medium heat until all the ingredients melt.

- ✓ Place the result into a blender and allow it to cool

- ✓ When you do this, blend the result until it is all thoroughly mixed (scrap the sides as you go).

- ✓ As you keep on blending, gently add the rose water to emulsify the mixture.

- ✓ Add also all the essential oil and blend quickly to incorporate them into the mixture.

- ✓ Add the cream into the glass jar and tightly cover it.

- ✓ Apply it daily on the abdomen to tighten the skin and reduce fat.

Chapter 4 – What to Look Out For When Buying Essential Oils?

It is vital that when you are buying essential oils, ensure that the bottle says '100% pure essential oil'. Also, make sure that the correct name of the species is well indicated in the label of the bottle.

If the word 'fragrance' is seen, have it in mind that there are almost always other additives.It is advisable that you buy essential oils from an organic source labelled as 'Therapeutic grade', this shows that they are toxin and additive free.

Therapeutic grades are undiluted and unfiltered. Be warned not to choose from Non-Genetically Modified Ingredients.

Conclusion

Closing Tips for Using Essential Oils to Achieve Your Weight Loss Goals

If you are a beginner to using essential oils, here are a few things that you should know to ease using them.

Firstly, it is advisable that if you are using essential oil as a newbie, ensure you do a body patch test on a small part of your skin (advisably your arm or leg) before you apply it on your whole body by rubbing or taking it directly internally. When you complete, whether you are allergic to an oil or not would be detected before you use a higher number of dosage.

Essential oils that pass this first quick skin patch test may be mildly irritating when you use them directly. You can also dilute your oil in a carrier oil like olive oil, coconut oil or jojoba oil before using it directly on your skin.

Ensure you limit the use of citrus-based oils (like orange and lemon essential oil) before using long period time outdoors, particularly during pool season and beach because they can be a cause of phototoxicity

Many oils are for external use only although it is not harmful if taken internally. But also make sure you get them fit for consumption before ingesting it.Lastly, always aim for the highest grade of essential oil that you can get.

Essential oils are implemented in various ways which are:

- ✓ capsules

- ✓ bath and body products

- ✓ massage oil

- ✓ diffusion

- ✓ rubs and balms

- ✓ inhalation

- ✓ food and drink recipes (when safe for internal use)

To achieve your weight loss goal, any of the recipes written above would apply. You can also take some recipes along with you to school, recreational activities, travel and work by making portable recipes. Your bracelet and necklace can be made with ceramic diffuser beads to hold the scent of your essential oil all day.

Essential oil isn't a miracle, they are only a push to your weight loss efforts. Don't stop your medication or prescription provided by your doctor. Using essential oil also shouldn't be a reason for living a reckless diet lifestyle.

Furthermore, problems such as depression, digestive disorder, autoimmune disorders, hypothyroidism and anxiety and other health and mood related issues associated with weight can be addressed using essential oils.

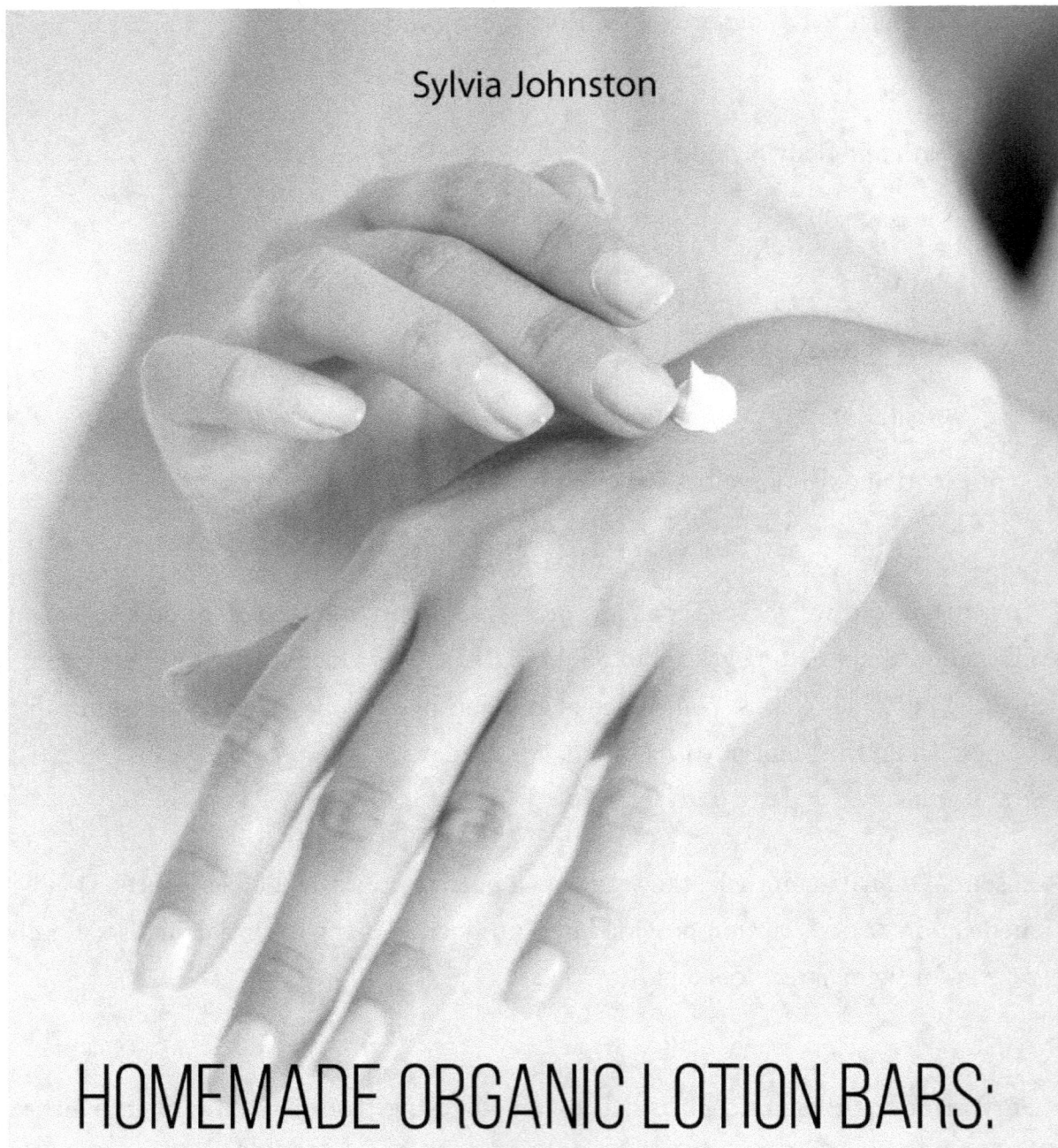

Sylvia Johnston

HOMEMADE ORGANIC LOTION BARS:

Natural Lotion Bars Recipes
Only from Non-Toxic Ingredients

Homemade Organic Lotion Bars:

Natural Lotion Bars Recipes Only from Non-Toxic Ingredients

Introduction: Quality that Can't Be Store Bought

Quality homemade bars of soap loaded with non-toxic all-natural ingredients such as lemon, citrus, and coconut are of a higher caliber than most of their store-bought brethren.

And drop in a few special oil-based compounds such as soybean oil, jasmine, or rosemary and you've got yourself a real winning combination. These DIY soaps cleanse as well as they soothe, and provide an unbeatable fragrance. All while providing you a way to cut off the daily bombardment of toxic chemicals that regular soap users are routinely exposed to.

So, if you are looking for a book to provide you with some wholesome soap recipes with all-natural ingredients, then look no further. Because this book, and the soap recipes herein, provide the kind of quality that just can't be store bought.

Chapter 1: Getting Your Soapy Supplies Ready

Soap making is a rich and rewarding experience but its only going to work if you have the right supplies. Besides the actual ingredients for your soap, you will need things like soap molds, protective gear, and appropriate cooking utensils. Here in this chapter we will give you a brief overview to get your soapy supplies ready!

Protective Goggles

As you work with soap it would be a good idea to where some sort of protective goggles. Although soap may seem like a tame enough material, there are chemicals involved, and any time you work with chemicals you run the risk of irritation to your eyes. Lye for example, can be particularly dangerous if it gets into your eyes.

The best way to avoid this danger is to simply make sure that your eyes are protected and covered at all times. They should be protected in this fashion during the whole process of soap making.

Work Gloves

As good as soap is you see, it is composed of a little something called "alkalies" and since these alkalies have a tremendous ability to dry out and dissolve oil based elements, being exposed to too much of it, or to a densely concentrated form can cause the skin to dry out or even break out into a rash

This is why it is necessary to take preventative measures such as this. Your hands are precious. They are the instruments with which you make your soap so you want to make sure that you protect them! In order to do so you will need to get some thick, industrial class work gloves.

Some may try to make soap with plastic or latex gloves, but these are not good options since borax and lye may eat right through them! Be sure to get some good work gloves!

Dust Mask

Making soap involves a lot of vapors and fumes, so unless you are exceptionally good at holding your breath—I would advise you to wear a protective dust mask. These small, but durable half masks, fit right on your face and serv to keep any wayward components of your soap from finding their way inside your respiratory tract!

And even if you do not suffer from devastating breathing difficulty there are many who have suffered through some pretty bad headaches from lingering fumes, so be sure to cover your face with a proper dust mask before making your soap.

Vinegar

If you have nothing else to use as a hardening agent, a little bit of vinegar could truly do some wonders. For anyone using vinegar, you will need to use just enough to offset the amount of oil that you use. The general rule is to make sure that you are able to replace water and oil with vinegar substrate.

If you do not want to use a whole lot of water, there are many recipes in which you could actually replace at least half of your H2O content with simple, plain old vinegar. As such, be sure to have a couple bottles of vinegar in stock.

Lye

While lye is most certainly not necessary when it comes to making natural soap, it doesn't hurt to have some on hand just in case you might need. Lye can almost be substituted for other oil-based ingredients but there are certain formulas that could use the kick that only lye could provide. Although not mandatory in its use, lye has been a part of soap making for quite a long time.

And there is a reason for its use as an ingredient. Lye is a great binding material and can really bring all of the elements of your soap ingredients together. Be sure to have this and all of the items, and supplies mentioned in this chapter on hand as you go about your soap making process.

Chapter 2: Medicinal and Cleansing Soap

No matter what may be ailing you—sometimes the best medicine you could ever be prescribed is simply a bar of soap that will get you nice and clean. Here in this chapter we provide you with several soapy examples that will do just that!

Almond Cleansing Soap

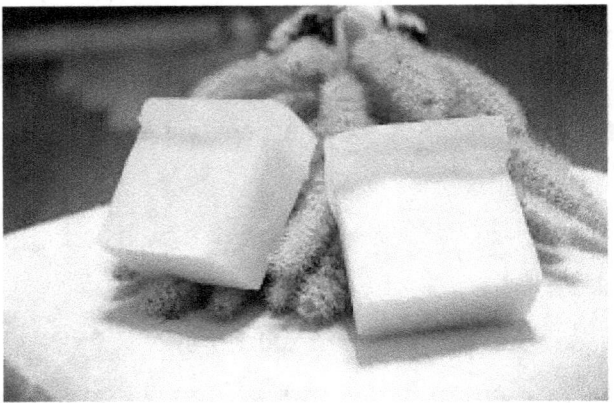

Almonds have a nourishing effect on skin and can bring moisture back to even the driest of surface layers. Almonds after all are full of Vitamin E and as such can provide some extra special protection from such things as the sun's grating rays. Almond soap also has vitamin A which is also quite good at clearing up just about any complexion.

Here are the exact ingredients:

16 ounces of palm oil

22 ounces of soybean oil

7 ounces of coconut oil

5 ounces of almond oil

3 cups of water

To begin, get out a large pot and add your 3 cups of water inside. Now set your stove for medium-high heat. Next, add your 5 ounces of almond oil, your 7 ounces of coconut oil, and your 22 ounces of soybean oil. Stir these a few minutes before adding in your 16 ounces of palm oil. Stir all of your ingredients together well and cook for 10 minutes.

After your ten minutes have passed, turn the stove off, and let the ingredients settle a moment, before you pour the contents of the pot inside the appropriate soap molds of your choosing. Allow the molds to dry out for 15 hours and your soaps are ready for use. You should have enough material to make several bars of soap with.

Organic Scalp Cleansing Soap

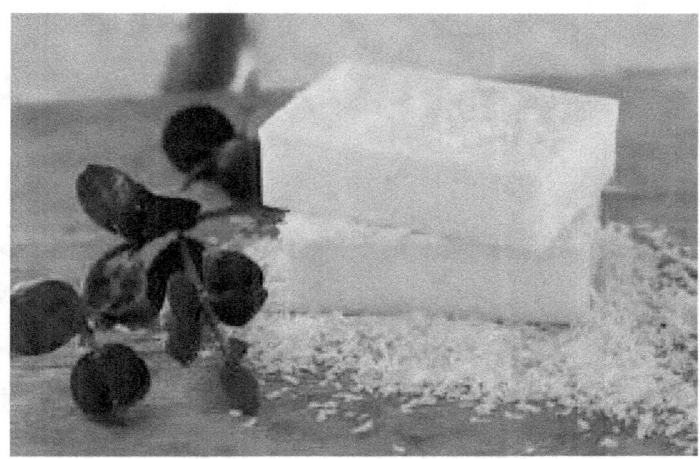

Do you ever have problems with greasy hair or dandruff? Are you looking for an all-natural, organic solution to your itchy scalp? Well then you should most certainly give this Organic Scalp Cleansing Soap a try!

I can remember times that my hair was so flaky I thought it was snowing every time I brushed it! But after just a few weeks of using this very special soap, my hair soon became free of dandruff and a whole lot less oily. This DIY soap delight is highly recommended.

Here are the exact ingredients:

3 ounces of lye

4 ounces of cocoa butter

4 ounces of coconut oil

3 ounces of castor oil

3 ounces of jojoba oil

3 ounces of Shea butter

2 ounces of beeswax

4 ounces of coconut milk

2 cups of water

First, get out a mixing bowl and deposit your 2 ounces of lye, your 2 cups of water, and your 4 ounces of coconut milk inside.Stir these ingredients together well before pouring them into a pan. Set your stove on medium-high heat and stir the ingredients continually over the next 15 to 20 minutes.

Now get out an additional mixing bowl and add your 2 ounces of beeswax, your 3 ounces of Shea butter, your 3 ounces of jojoba oil, your 3 ounces of castor oil, and your 4 ounces of coconut oil. Stir these ingredients together well and put the mixing bowl in the microwave on high heat for about 30 seconds. The ingredients should melt and meld together well.

After this, dump the melted mixing bowl ingredients into the pan on the stove, stir everything together and cook on medium-high heat for another few minutes.

Finally, pour the cooked ingredients into your soap molds and let them dry and solidify within the mold for 15 hours.

The Veggie Cleanser

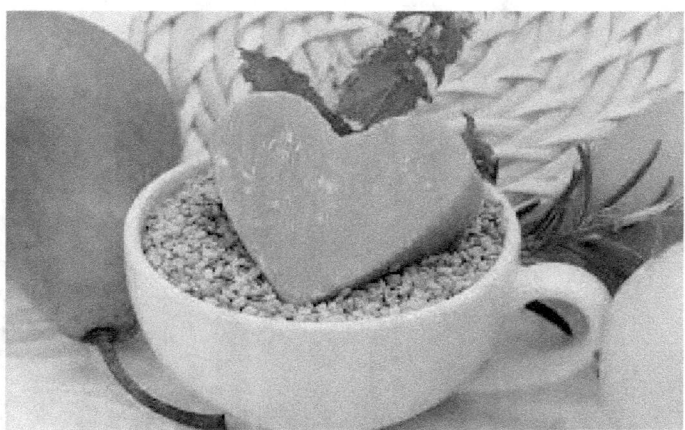

Remember when your folks told you to eat your vegetables? Well what about washing with them? Vegetable soap? Who would have thought right?But as it turns out the vegetable extracts in this soap bar make for the perfect cleanser! The vitamins and nutrients in this soap are just perfect for rebuilding degenerative tissue of the skin. This is regenerative (and clean) medicine at its best!

Here are the exact ingredients:

18 ounces of carrot juice

20 ounces of coconut oil

18 ounces of canola oil

18 ounces of vegetable oil

20 ounces of olive oil

3 cups of water

To begin, place a pot on the stove, set the temp for medium-high and then add your 3 cups of water to the pot. After this add your 18 ounces of carrot juice followed by your 20 ounces of coconut oil, your 18 ounces of canola oil, your 18 ounces of vegetable oil, and your 20 ounces of olive oil.

Now stir everything together as it cooks over the next 15 to 20 minutes. Finally, take your cooked ingredients and pour them into some molds. Allow them to harden for about 10 hours before use.

Medicinal Lavender

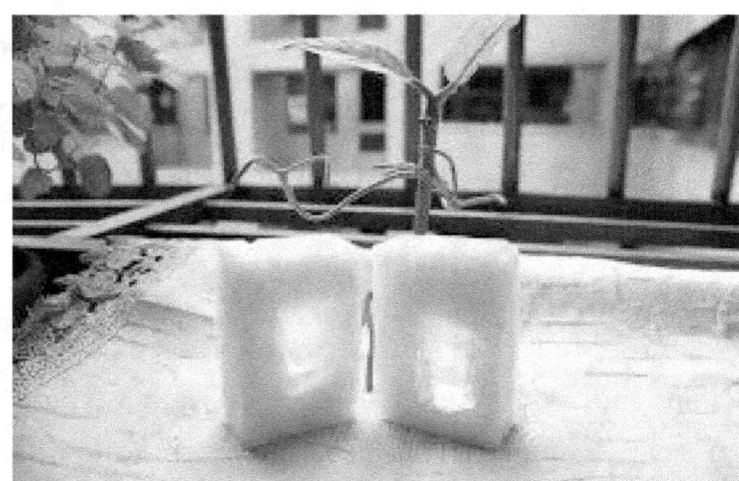

Lavender has many medicinal properties such as being able to ease inflammation. As such, this soap can work wonders for someone who has broken out into a rash.

I can personally vouch for this due to a run in with some poison ivy earlier this spring. I was doing some yard work when I came into contact with the toxic plant and both of my arms broke out as a result.But by scrubbing away at the inflamed skin with some good old Medicinal Lavender I was able to take much of the sting out of the poison ivy rash and speed up my recovery.

If you are having skin issues, you never have to suffer in silence again. Just make this soap bar and make it a part of your daily routine. You'll be glad that you did. This soap is highly recommended.

Here are the exact ingredients:

1 ounce of almond oil

1 ounce of palm oil

1 ounce of coconut oil

4 ounces of lavender oil

2 ounces of olive oil

3 cups of milk

1 cup of water

Get out a pot and place it onto a stove set for high heat. Now add your 3 cups of milk and 1 cup of water to the pot. This should then be followed by your ounce of almond oil, your ounce of palm oil, your ounce of coconut oil, and your 2 ounces of olive oil.

Briefly stir these ingredients before adding your 4 ounces of lavender oil. Now mix it all up and allow to cook for about 30 minutes. After this pour the mixture directly into your molds and have them solidify and dry out over the next 10 hours.

Chapter 3: Non-Toxic Cosmetic Soap

There are a lot of toxins in our normal everyday environment, and surprisingly many of the store-bought soaps, shampoos, and deodorants have more than their fair share of toxins as well. It does seem rather ironic that we would lather up and wash ourselves with something that contains toxins, but this is actually standard fare for most.

Having that said, it's really no wonder people have dry skin, flaky, dandruff filled hair, and inflamed armpits. In order to break away from this detrimental routine, here in this chapter we present to you some of the best DIY recipes for non-toxic cosmetic soap.

Banana Boat Soap

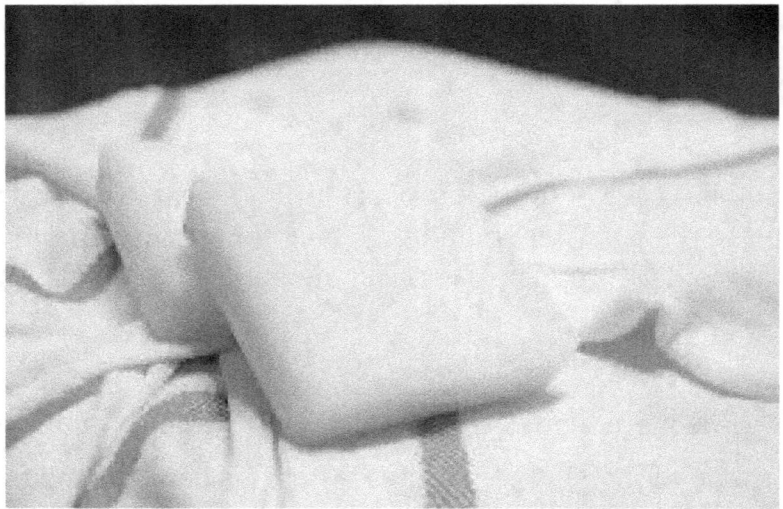

You like Bananas? Then you are going to love this soap! This banana-based soap does a tremendous job of moisturizing and cleansing your skin. It's a dual-purpose workhorse of clean goodness at your disposal.

The main ingredient of this soap—potassium hydroxide—is excellent at evenly distributing moisture throughout the cells of the skin as well as balancing out the entire PH level of the dermis.

Here are the exact ingredients:

4 ounces of borax

5 ounces of potassium hydroxide

5 ounces of coconut oil

10 ounces of olive oil

2 cups of water

To get started, get out a large pot and place it on a stove adjusted for medium-high heat. Now add your 2 cups of water to the pot and wait a few minutes until the water comes to a boil.

Once the water is beginning to boil you can then add your 4 ounces of borax, your 5 ounces of potassium hydroxide, your 5 ounces of coconut oil, and your 10 ounces of olive oil. Stir all of these ingredients together well for about 15 minutes.

Once your 15 minutes have passed you can then pour your ingredients into your waiting soap molds and allow them to solidify into hard bars of soap over the next 10 hours.

Exfoliating Lemon Bar

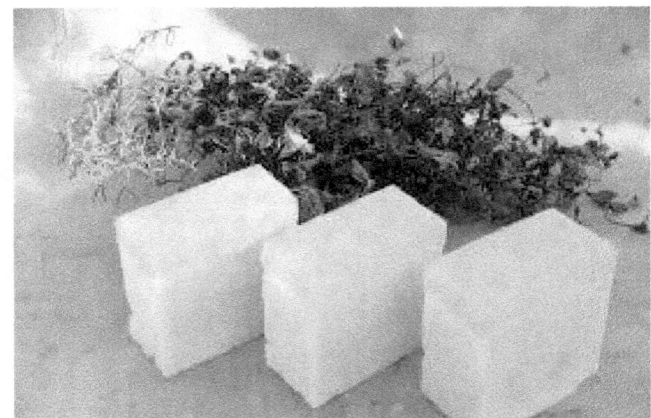

Have you ever noticed how so many cleaning products from laundry detergent to dish soap are either "lemon scented" or otherwise have lemon as a main ingredient? There is indeed a reason for this Lemon you see, is a natural cleaning agent. This soap cleans, exfoliates, and leaves you with a fresh lemony scent! And this soap in particular is fantastic at scraping away the grime and leaving you clean and fresh!

Here are the exact ingredients:

11 ounces of lemon juice

1 ounce of lemon oil

1 cup of water

1 cup of milk

In order to create your own exfoliating lemon bar, you will need to get out a large pot and add your cup of water and your cup of milk to the pot. Stir these ingredients together for a few minutes and allow to come to a boil.

After this, you can then add your 11 ounces of lemon juice, and your ounce of lemon oil. Stir these ingredients together well over the course of the next 8 to 10 minutes. Once thoroughly mixed and cooked, you can then pour the mixture into soap molds. Allow the soaps to solidify over the next 10 hours.

Orange Face Soap

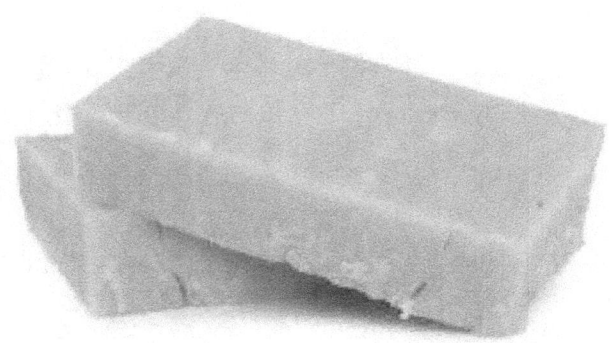

Despite what the Oompa Loompas may have told you this soap doesn't mean you'll have an orange face after using it! The soap itself is made out of orange juice, along with special infused oils, and cocoa butter. Orange juice is a natural exfoliating and the exfoliating element that it provides in this soap is nothing short of tremendous.

This soap can naturally rejuvenate the skin and provide relief from blemishes. If for example you are suffering from acne, or even eczema—this soap could be of tremendous help in your recovery. Oranges are a medicinal food that help boost our immune system and they provide relief to inflammation. This soap is a real winner. You are really going to love it!

Here are the exact ingredients:

12 ounces of orange juice

1 ounce of orange oil

5 ounces of olive oil

4 ounces of cocoa butter

2 cups of water

Orange bar soap is great for the skin and is as nourishing as it is enriching. In order to create your own orange bar soap fill cup a large pot with 2 cups of water and place it on a stove set for medium-high heat.

Next, add your 12 ounces of orange juice, your ounce of orange oil, your 5 ounces of olive oil and your 4 ounces of cocoa butter. Stir and cook these ingredients over the next 10 minutes. Once your 10 minutes have passed you can then pour your soap mixture into your soap molds and leave them out to dry for about 15 hours.

Palm Kernel Shave Cream Soap

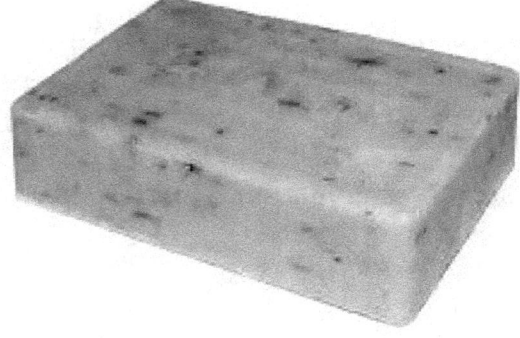

Palm Kernel Shave Cream Soap! Good for your face, arms, legs, armpits—or whatever else you may have to shave! The all-natural chemistry of this soap really comes together to create a smooth glide for your razor blade. With this mixture of coconut and palm kernel, it's always a real pleasure to lather up for a close shave.

Here are the exact ingredients:

10 ounces of palm kernel oil

10 ounces of olive oil

5 ounces of coconut oil

1 cup of water

To produce this rich soap, start off with a medium sized pan and a cup of water. Next, add in your 10 ounces of palm kernel oil and your 10 ounces of olive oil followed by your 5 ounces of coconut oil.

Stir these ingredients together well as they cook over the next 5 minutes. Once thoroughly mixed together you can then pour the mix into your soap molds. Allow to harden for at least 8 hours before use.

Chapter 4: Soap for Your Pets

Anyone who has a cat or dog know just how difficult grooming your animals can be. They don't like the water, and they don't like the soap. They would rather be anywhere but where you are when it's for them to wash up.

But washing your pets does not have to be a terrible chore. The homemade soaps presented in this chapter provide a tremendous resource to all of your pet cleaning efforts. If you need a good soap for your pet feel free to try them all.

Dog Gone Soap

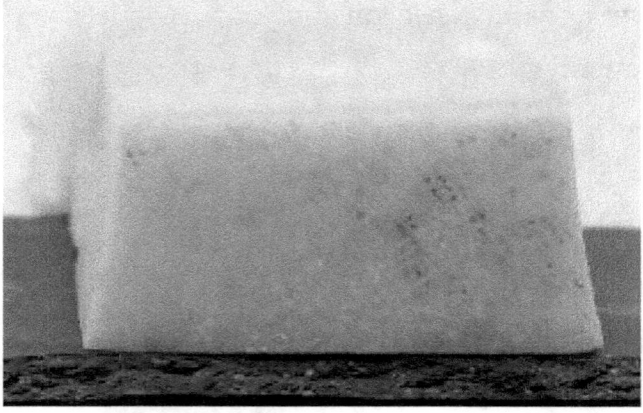

If your doggie needs a good soap to get him up and going. You might want to give this one a try. It's loaded with soybean and olive oil. This recipe creates just the right mixture to keep the moisture in your dog's scalp but out of its hair. This soap is also a tremendous oil fighter, providing your dog with a great clean coat of fur.

Here are the exact ingredients:

3 ounces of soybean oil

3 ounces of olive oil

3 ounces of coconut oil

3 ounces of avocado oil

4 ounces of rosemary oil

1 ounce of lye

2 cups of water

Put your 2 cups of water into a pot, followed by your ounce of lye. Set the stove for high heat. Now stir the ingredients together as they cook a few minutes before adding in your 3 ounces of avocado oil.

Stir these together briefly and then add your 3 ounces of soybean oil, your 3 ounces of olive oil, and your 4 ounces of rosemary oil. Stir and cook these ingredients together for another few minutes. Once everything is mixed and cooked, pour ingredients into soap molds and allow to settle in place for about 8 hours. After this, the soap is ready for use.

Kitty Cat Bar

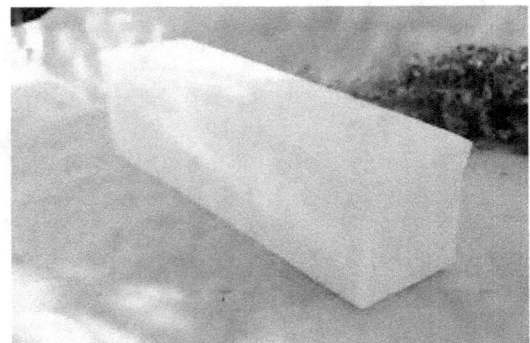

This is some pretty heavy-duty soap for your cat. It's composed primarily of Shea butter, giving it a very smooth sheen. If your cat needs an extra shine to its coat you may want to give this Kitty Cat Bar a try.

Here are the exact ingredients:

4 ounces of Shea butter

4 ounces of beeswax

4 ounces of coconut oil

2 cups of water

Place a large pot onto a stove set for high heat and then add your 2 cups of water. After your water has been added you can then go ahead and add your 4 ounces of Shea butter, your 4 ounces of beeswax, and your 4 ounces of coconut oil.

Stir these ingredients together as they cook over the next few minutes. Turn burner off and allow ingredients to settle in place for a moment before pouring the mixture into your molding. Allow soap mixture to solidify and harden in the soap molds for about 8 hours before use.

Flea and Tick Proof Soap

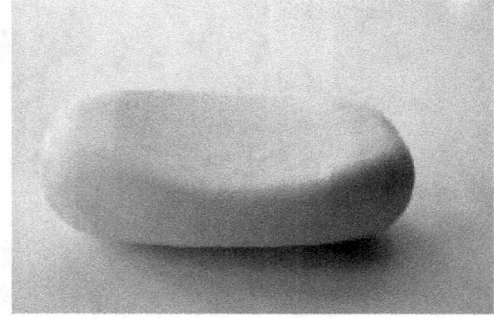

Tick season is terrible this year. I can attest to that myself. The other day I was out in the back of my property walking my dog when I noticed a tick right on top of the little guy's head. It thankfully hadn't attached yet so I went to knock it off. Right after knocking this tick off I then noticed another one crawling on my arm!

I think both me and my dog both were ready to run inside at that point! But the best way to beat the ticks this season is simply to stay as clean as possible. After your dog comes in from a long excursion outdoors wash him down with this flea and tick proof soap and those critters won't stand a chance.

Here are the exact ingredients:

3 cups of cinnamon oil

3 cups of thyme

3 cups of clove oil

4 cups of rosemary

3 cups of beeswax

3 cups of mango butter

1 cup of coconut oil

2 cups of water

To get started, deposit your 2 cups of water into a pot and set the stove for high heat. Now add your 3 cups of cinnamon oil, your 3 cups of thyme, your 3 cups of clove oil, your 4 cups of rosemary, your 3 cups of beeswax, your 3 cups of mango butter, and your cup of coconut oil.

Stir everything together well as they cook over the course of the next ten minutes. After this, pour the mixture into your molds and allow them to harden for the next 10 hours. Once hardened, use when ready.

Furry Friend Fragrance

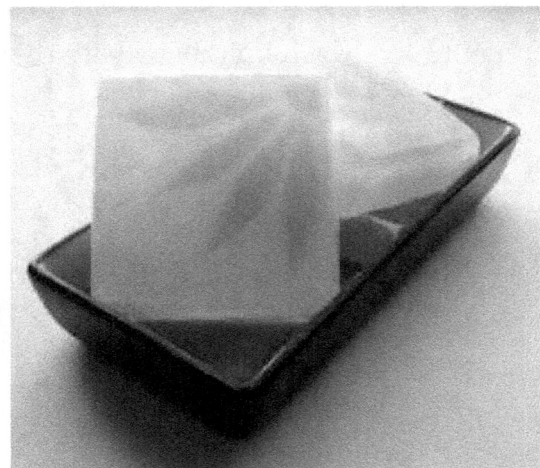

If your little doggy has been smelling kind of funny lately, you just might want to give him a little bit of help in the odor apartment.

Many dog soaps simply mask the odor but the great thing about this fragrant bit of soap is that it neutralizes the odor at the source as well as leaving a fragrant aroma behind in its wake. Don't let your dog stink! Give him the Furry Friend Fragrance he needs!

Here are the exact ingredients:

3 ounces of citronella

3 ounces of sweet orange essential oil

5 ounces of coconut oil

14 ounces of olive oil

5 ounces of lye

2 cups of water

Making this soap is a breeze. Simply get out a large pot, place onto a stove at medium-high heat, and add your 2 cups of water. After this, you can then add your 3 ounces of citronella, your 3 ounces of sweet orange essential oil, your 5 ounces of coconut oil, your 14 ounces of olive oil, and finally your 5 ounces of lye.

Stir these ingredients together well over the course of the next 20 minutes. Once cooked allow to settle in the pot for a moment before pouring into your molding. Keep the soap mixture inside your molding for about 10 hours. Once hard and dry, this soap is ready for use.

Chapter 5: Uniquely Made Soap Creations

Have you ever heard of soap made out of Dr. Pepper? What about beer? Yes, sometimes it seems that soap can be literally made out of just about anything, and here in this chapter we show you some truly unique homemade soap creations.

The Budweiser Bar

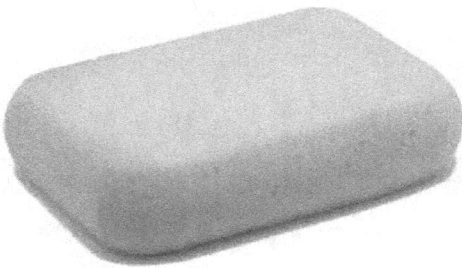

Rather than drinking Budweiser at the bar why not take a bat with a Budweiser bar of soap! Before you think this is absolutely batty just consider the fact that beer is a great cleanser and exfoliant for the skin!

Yep, that's right! Studies have actually proven that the hops component of common, everyday beer is full of all kinds of enriching amino acids that make the skin smooth and soft!

Beer actually has a lot of skin healthy vitamins as well, making it an all-around skin friendly cocktail of ingredients! And don't worry—this soap won't keep you from driving home afterwards!

Here are the exact ingredients:

30 ounces of Budweiser

10 ounces of olive oil

10 ounces of coconut oil

1 cup of water

In order to make your own Budweiser soap, get out a large pot, put it on a stove set for medium-high heat and add your cup of water. Next add your 30 ounces of Budweiser, followed by your 10 ounces of olive oil, and your 10 ounces of coconut oil.

Stir these ingredients together well over the next 10 minutes. Turn your stove off and allow the mixture to settle for a minute or so. After this, you can then pour the mixture into your molding. Keep inside the soap molds for at least 8 hours. They should now be solid and ready for use.

Soda Bar Soap

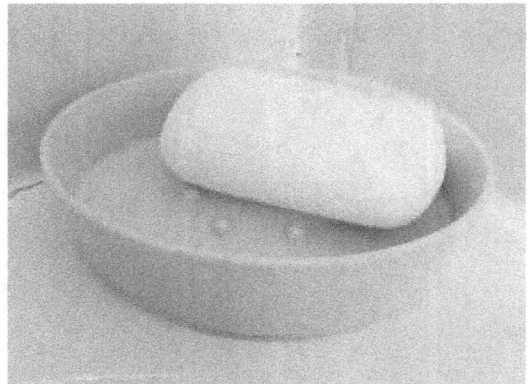

Would you like to try some soda soap? No—we're not talking baking soda here—we're talking soda soda! Made from any variety of soda-based beverage you could imagine, this novelty soap is not only unique, it actually cleans pretty good too! Even while allowing you to smell like grape soda! Isn't life great?

Here are the exact ingredients:

20 ounces of a soda-based beverage

10 ounces of lemon juice

2 ounces of borax

2 cups of water

Get out a large cooking pot and add your 2 cups of water before setting the stovetop burner to medium heat. Now add your 20 ounces of soda (Dr. Pepper, Pepsi, any beverage you like), followed by your 10 ounces of lemon juice, and your 2 ounces of borax. Take especial care to keep the borax out of your eyes, as it can cause irritation.

Stir everything together well and cook for about 3 to 5 minutes. After this, let the mixture settle a bit before pouring into your soap molds. Keep the mixture in the soap molds over the next 8 to 10 hours. They should now be ready to be pried out of the molding. Use whenever you are ready to do so.

Spicy Soap

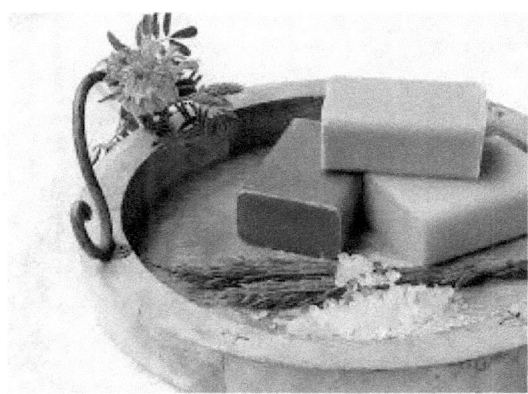

If you want to add some spice in your nice and cleanly life, add this Spicy Soap to your bath time regimen! This soap dares to include 10 full ounces of habanero oil. Habanero oil you see is full of a little something called curcumin. Curcumin is good for us in a wide variety of ways from fighting inflammation to slowing down our metabolism.

In soap form it is its inflammation fighting power that is the most promising. Just lather up some of this skin on an arm broken out in a rash and soon enough that arm will be as clear as the day you were born! This soap is also an excellent exfoliant and quite good at clearing up acne. Go ahead and give this Spicy Soap a try! You will most certainly be glad that you did!

Here are the exact ingredients:

10 ounces of habanero oil

2 ounces of mango butter

5 ounces of olive oil

5 ounces of coconut oil

2 ounces of lye

1 cup of water

Place a large pot onto your stovetop and set the burner on high. Add your cup of water followed by your 10 ounces of habenero oil, your 2 ounces of mango butter, your 5 ounces of olive oil, your 5 ounces of coconut oil, and your 2 ounces of lye.

Stir everything together well over the course of the next 5 to 10 minutes. Once the mixture has been cooked allow to settle for a moment, and then pour it all out inside of your soap moldings. Keep in moldings for at least 8 hours before use.

Strawberry and Cream Bar

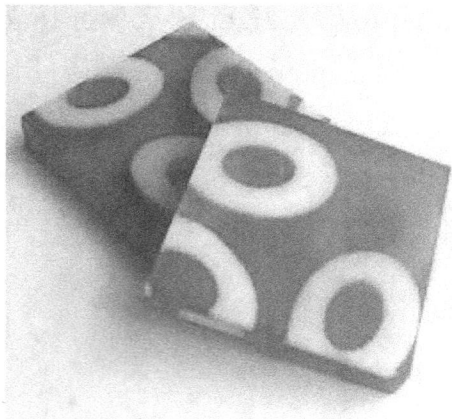

It's like desert decided to pay your bath time routine a visit! What can I say? If you like strawberries and cream then you are going to love this bar of soap! It's more than just a novel luxury however, this soap can really clean and detox your skin!

Strawberry juice is known to slow the aging process of our skin, fighting wrinkles and evening out our skin tone when we get older. The combination of strawberry and coconut are also powerful in antioxidants, greatly boosting the elastic integrity of our dermis. Try this soap today!

Here are the exact ingredients:

7 ounces of strawberry juice

2 ounces of sodium hydroxide

5 ounces of palm oil

5 ounces of coconut oil

3 ounces of lye

2 cups of water

This most certainly is an interesting batch of soap. In order to create your own version—here's what you have to do. Get out a large pot and place it onto a stovetop burner set for high heat. Next, add your 2 cups of water followed by your 7 ounces of strawberry juice, your 2 ounces of sodium hydroxide, your 5 ounces of coconut oil, and your 3 ounces of lye.

Stir everything together well before allowing to settle for 2 or 3 minutes. Finally, pour the mix into your soap molds and let harden for 8 to 10 hours. Once hard and dry, this soap is ready for use!

Conclusion: Where there is Hope—There is Soap!

We see our soap in the soap dish or hanging at the corner rim of our bath tub and not think much of it. But without soap life would be pretty miserable, pretty quickly. Just think of the last time that you really needed nothing more than a hot shower and a good bar of soap.

Maybe you just got back from a long day at work or you were working hard out in the yard—either way, when you were done you knew that nothing would quite make you feel better other than cleaning and refreshing that outside layer we commonly call our skin, with a nice bar of soap.

Soap cleanses, refreshes and heals. And as such, many varieties of soap with many purported purposes have been created throughout the years. Here in this book we have presented to you quite a wide variety of soap types which all have a multiplicity of uses I really do hope that you have find the tips, recipes, and advice in this book helpful.

And if you follow the guidelines of this book as presented to you, I know that this hope is not in vain. Because where there is hope after all—there is soap!

Thank you for reading! And good luck!